Grandpa Remembers Love

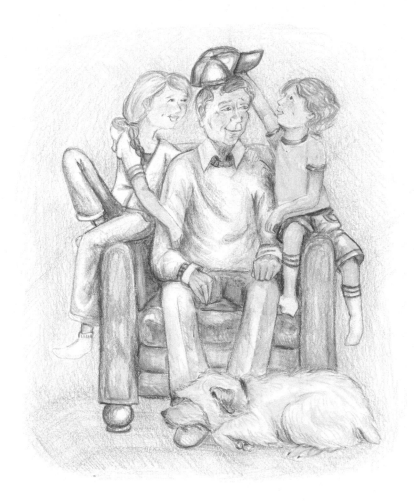

Written by Theresa Matocha LCSW, CDP
Illustrations by Lillian Stein

AuthorHouse™
1663 Liberty Drive
Bloomington, IN 47403
www.authorhouse.com
Phone: 833-262-8899

Because of the dynamic nature of the Internet, any web addresses or links contained in this book may have changed since publication and may no longer be valid. The views expressed in this work are solely those of the author and do not necessarily reflect the views of the publisher, and the publisher hereby disclaims any responsibility for them.

Any people depicted in stock imagery provided by Getty Images are models, and such images are being used for illustrative purposes only.
Certain stock imagery © Getty Images.

This book is printed on acid-free paper.

ISBN: 978-1-4490-8695-4 (sc)

Print information available on the last page.

Published by AuthorHouse 02/03/2023

authorHOUSE®

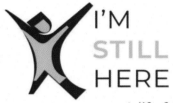

I'M
STILL
HERE

A life fulfilling approach to living with dementia

A portion of the proceeds from the sale of this book will be donated to the *I'm Still Here Foundation.* Their mission:

I'm Still Here (ISH) helps people living with dementia to flourish through engagement in life, family and community. ISH supports programs that engage persons living with dementia and their care partners in arts, culture and community. ISH seeks to spread the message of hope and possibility, especially to underserved individuals and communities.

Learn more at: www.imstillhere.org

For grandparents and parents living with memory loss and the children who love them.

To Fausto…who will always be my brother!

Special thanks to:

Paige Ackerson-Kiley, MFA and Barbara McKay, MA
For their artistic and professional guidance.

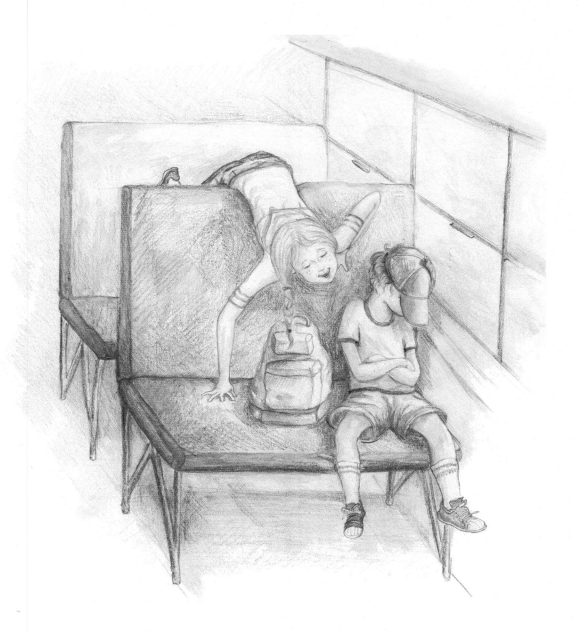

"Grandma's going to tell us something special about Grandpa
Jack today!" Elaine excitedly reminded her little brother Teddy
as she hopped onto the school bus.

As the children settled into their seat, Elaine noticed Teddy had pulled his baseball cap over his eyes. She knew this usually meant he was upset about something.

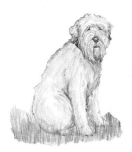

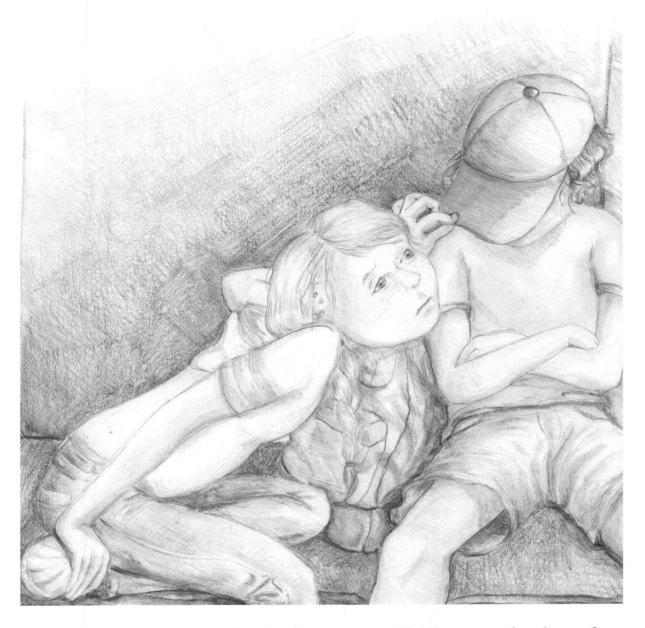

"Hey Teddy Bear, what's the matter?" Elaine asked as she peeked under his cap.

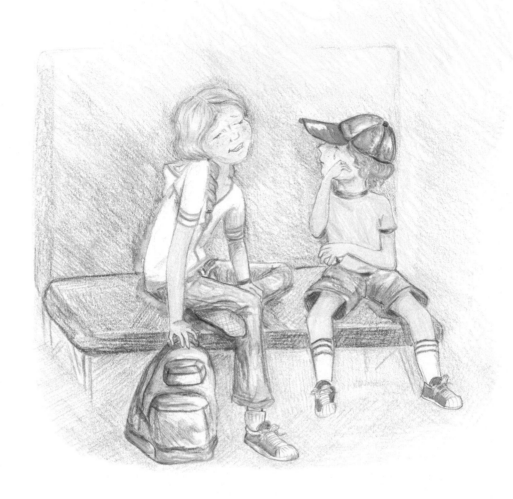

Teddy looked at Elaine through tear-filled eyes. "I'm scared to see Grandpa today—he doesn't know my name anymore and he looks mad when I ask him to play catch with me." "He can't help it, Teddy—Grandpa has something wrong with his memory. It's nothing to be scared about. Think about Grandma's homemade snacks and you'll feel better."

4

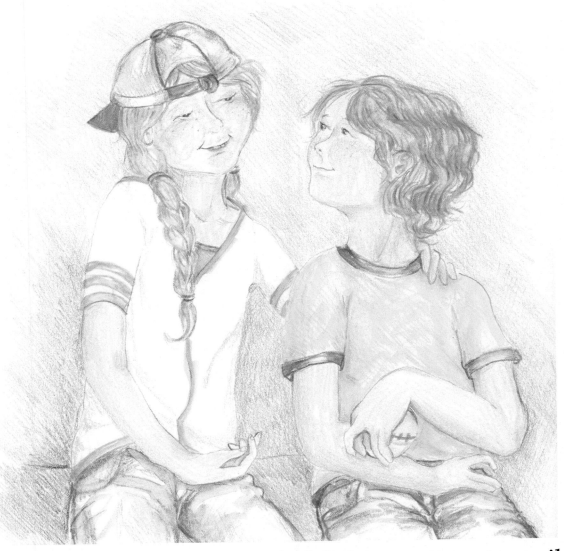

The thought of Grandma Mary's delicious treats put a smile on Teddy's face. He decided to keep his fingers crossed that Grandpa Jack might play catch with him today.

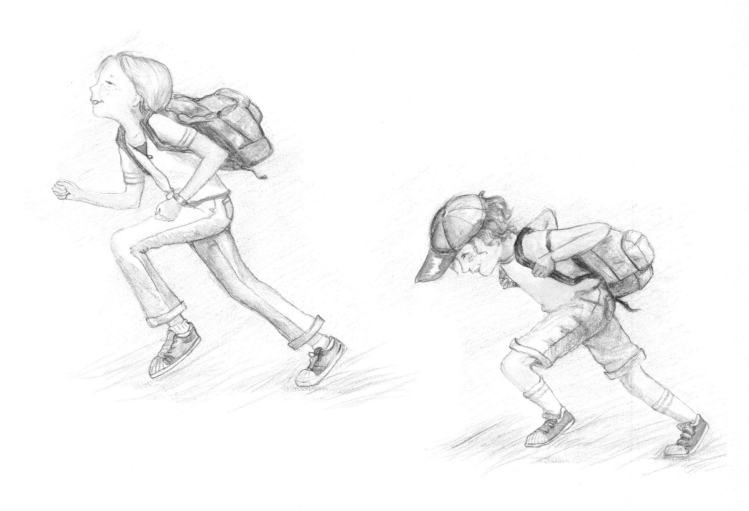

When the bus pulled up to Grandpa Jack and Grandma Mary's house, the children gathered their backpacks, hurried off and ran up to the back door by the kitchen.

As always, Grandma Mary had a big hug waiting for them. "Thank goodness for Thursday afternoons! I look forward to this hug all week long!" Even though Grandma said the same thing every week, the children never grew tired of hearing it.

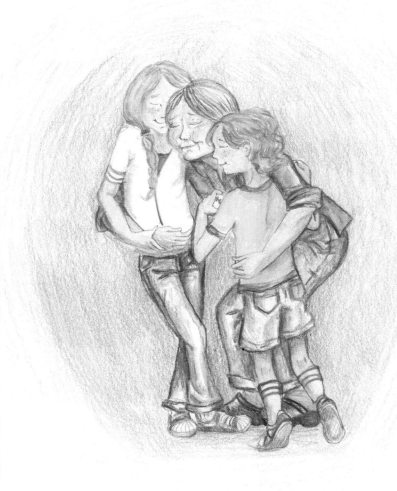

"How about some fresh-out-of-the-oven apple turnovers for my fresh-out-of-school grandchildren?" "Yes, Please!" Elaine and Teddy said eagerly. "Well then," said Grandma, "let's wash those hands and it will be my pleasure to serve you."

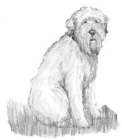

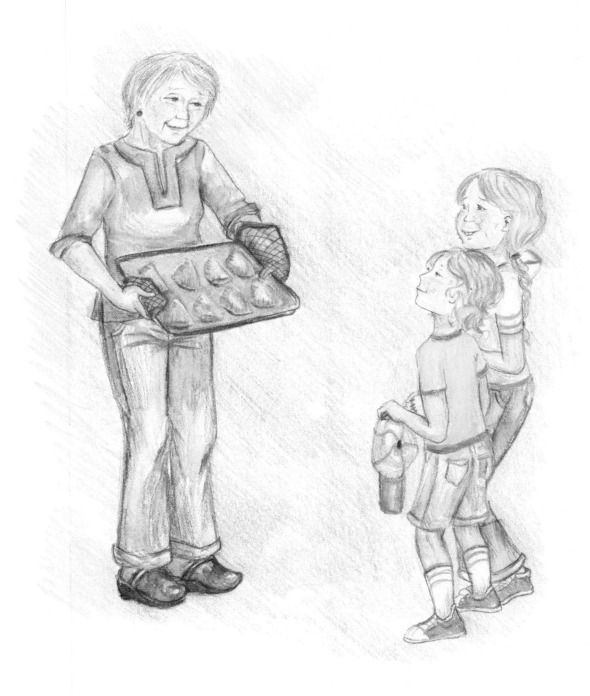

As the children enjoyed their turnovers, loud snoring sounds drifted in from the living room.

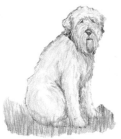

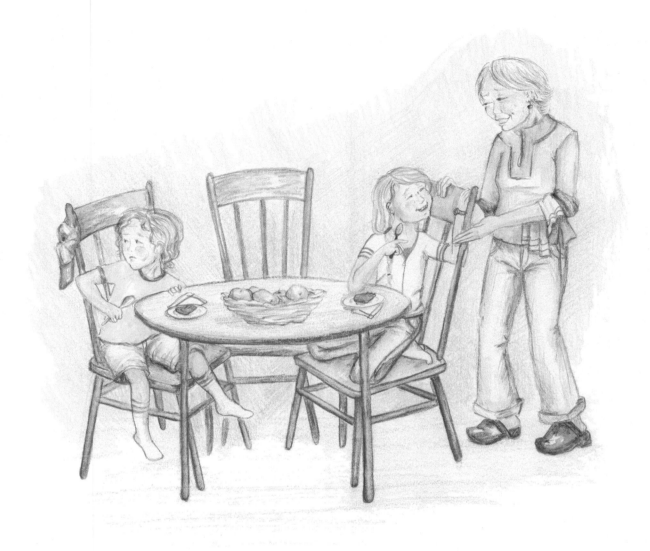

"We called that noise sawing wood when I was a little girl!"
Grandma grinned. "Grandpa sure can saw wood while he's
taking a nap!" Elaine said. "Believe it or not," said Grandma, "I
can sleep right through that saw after fifty years of snuggling
with your Grandpa!"

"Which reminds me, I promised to tell you something special about Grandpa Jack today." "Yes! Yes! You did! What is it Grandma?"

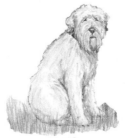

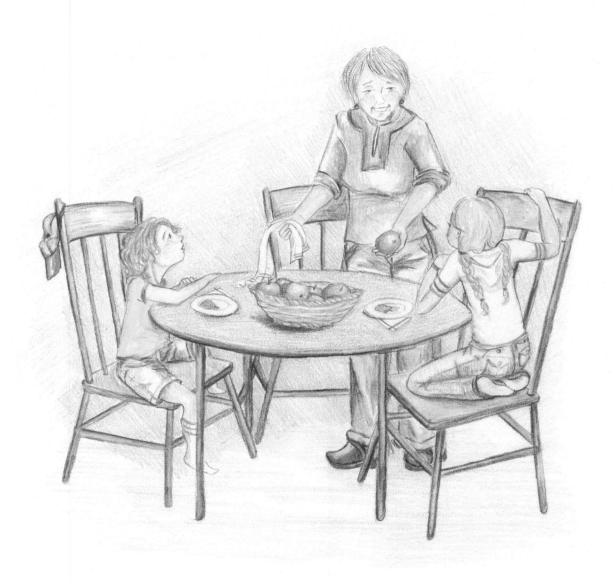

"Well, you know your Grandfather has been forgetting a lot of things for a while now. Things that seem simple for us—like what to do with a towel or the name of a type of food. But sometimes he *can* remember things that happened a long time ago."

"But Grandma, we already *know* that. He doesn't even remember our *names* anymore but he tells stories about being a little boy. How can he remember that far back and not know who we are!?" Elaine was confused.

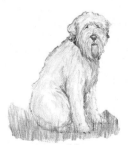

14

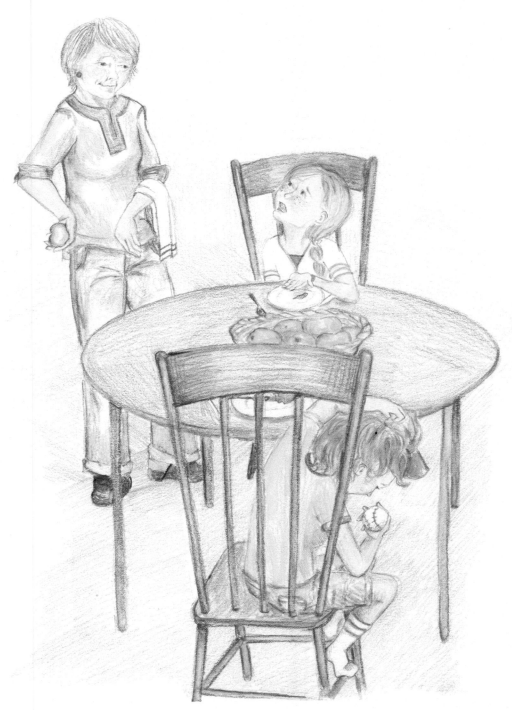

Teddy pulled his baseball cap over his eyes and Grandma sat down beside him. "What are you thinking about, Teddy?" Grandma asked. "I miss the way Grandpa used to be. He won't throw the baseball around with me anymore." "It's not that he doesn't want to play catch with you, Teddy." Grandma explained. "He just needs some help getting started."

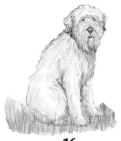

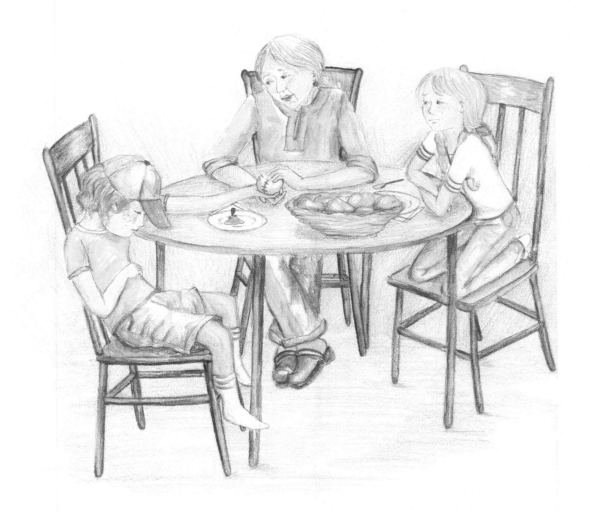

"Answering questions is hard for Grandpa right now. Instead of *asking* him to play catch you could try putting his baseball mitt into his hand *for* him, and tossing the ball *to* him. There's a good chance he'll still know what to do with that ball because it's something he learned to do a long time ago."

"But why does Grandpa *look* the same? And he's still so strong! How can he see and hear things but not remember anything, Grandma?" asked Teddy. "Well, sometimes when we get older our brains don't work as well as our bodies" Grandma explained. "Does Grandpa know he can't remember things?" Elaine asked. "Not any more dear. There was a time when he did know and he understood that his memory could get worse."

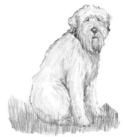

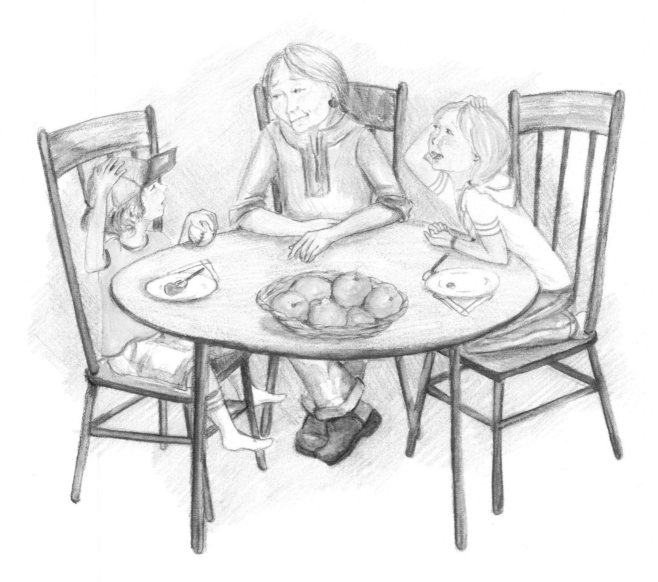

"Grandpa has something called 'dementia' which means he can't make memories the way he used to. " Will Grandpa's memory ever come back into his head?" Teddy asked. "No Teddy, not in the way we wish it could."

19

Grandma Mary warmly wrapped her arms around her grandchildren and said: "Here's the special thing I want you to know: Grandpa, remembers love."

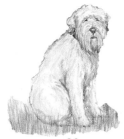

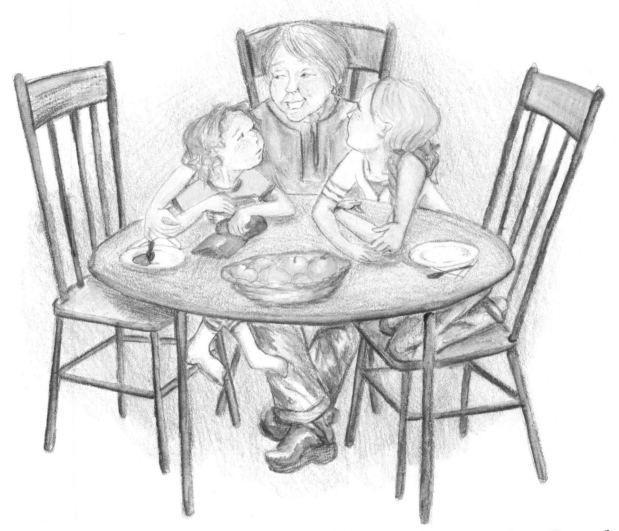

"What do you mean Grandma?" "Well, you know that Grandpa
Jack smiles and laughs and even cries sometimes. That's
because he still has feelings. That part of him has not gone
away."

"Have you seen the happy look on his face when we walk around our garden? He loves smelling the flowers and touching the growing vegetables—even though he can't garden himself anymore."

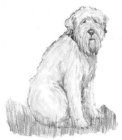

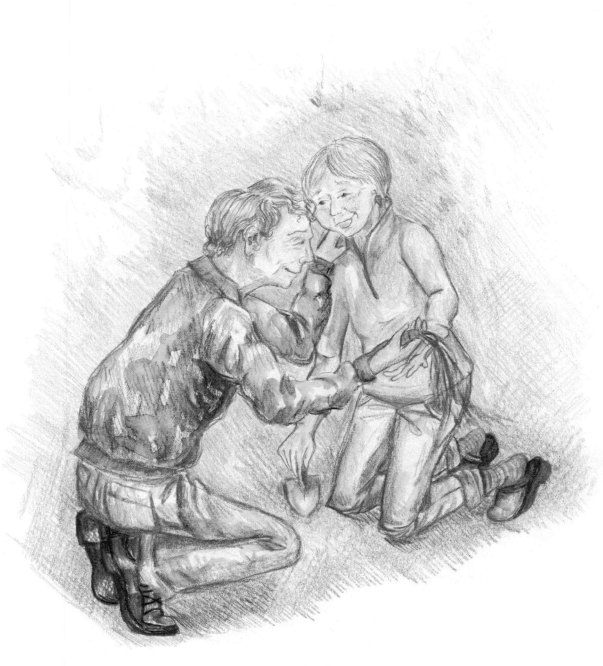

"Remember when Grandpa was sad because he couldn't figure out how to tie his shoes and Ruffles cheered him up with a big doggie kiss?"

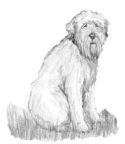

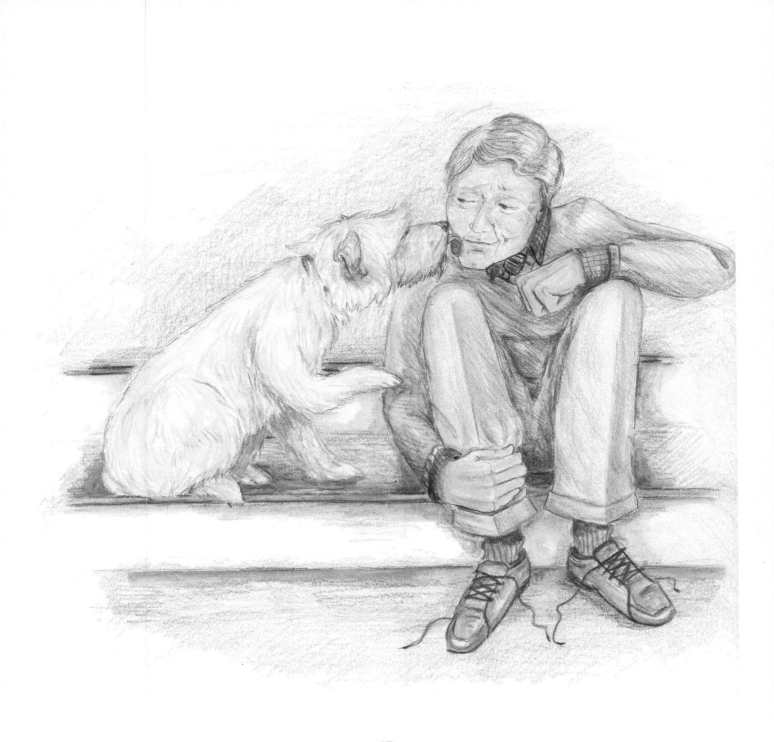

"Sometimes, when I take the blanket off the sofa and wrap it around him while he's resting, he leans over to give me a kiss. But he doesn't know how to say 'thank-you' anymore. That's what I mean."

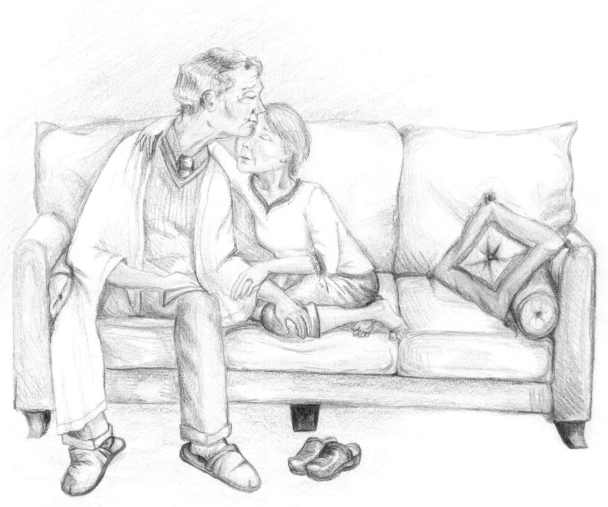

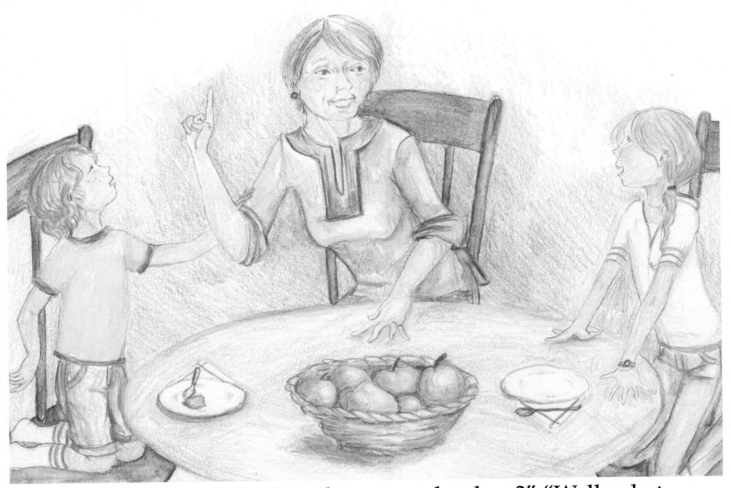

"How can we help Grandpa remember love?" "Well, what makes you feel loved?" Grandma asked. "How about making a list—it would give you ideas for helping Grandpa." Elaine and Teddy excitedly grabbed some paper and pencils and started their lists.

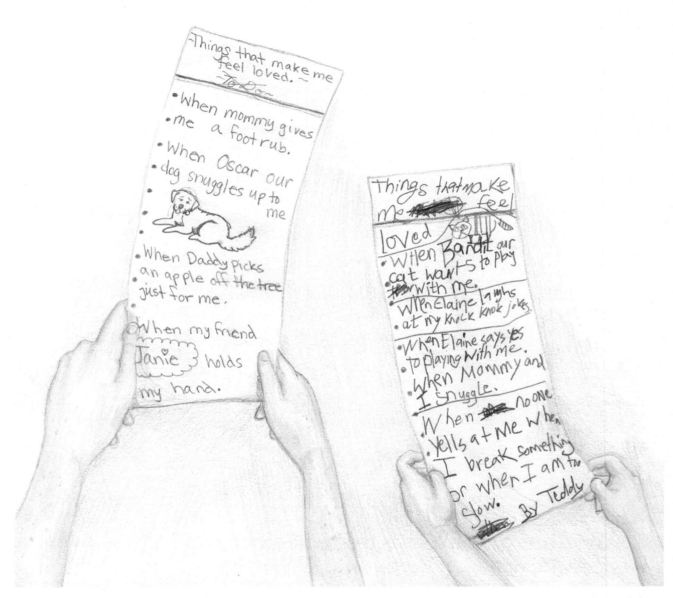

Grandma looked at what the children had written and smiled.
"These are wonderful lists! I think Grandpa Jack would love all
of these things too."

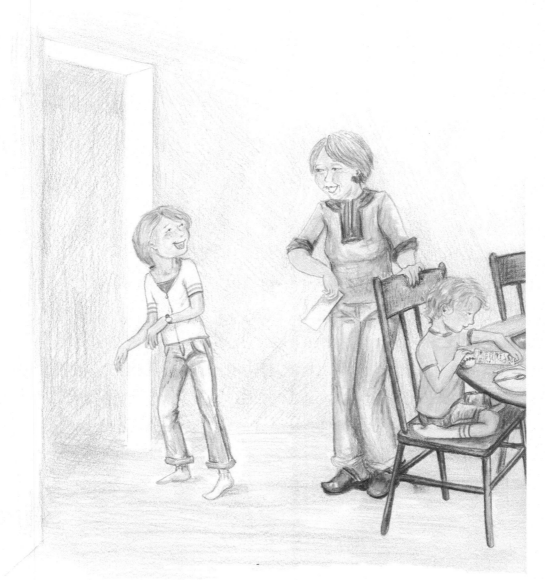

"Can I try out my ideas right now?" Elaine anxiously asked. "I haven't heard that saw running for a while now!" Grandma said with a grin. Elaine wasted no time dashing into the living room to see Grandpa Jack.

Grandma turned back toward Teddy who was staring at his list. "Grandma, you said Grandpa Jack remembers love, but I want to help him remember baseball because I know it's something *he* loves. Is that the same thing?" "Yes, Teddy," Grandma nodded. "How can I do it Grandma?" "Well, let me think about that one for a minute," Grandma said.

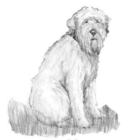

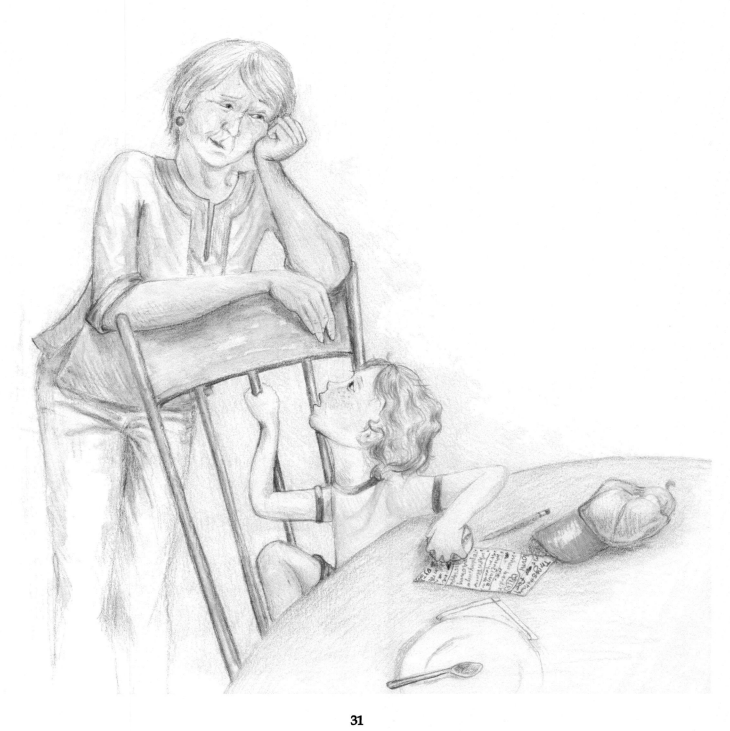

"You know Teddy, Grandpa loved reading baseball stories. I know you are working on your reading skills at school—what if you read Grandpa a story from one of his baseball books? There's nothing wrong with his hearing!"

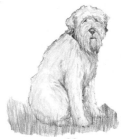

"I can do that Grandma! I know just what story I want to read to him!" Teddy practically flew toward Grandpa's bookshelf he was so excited.

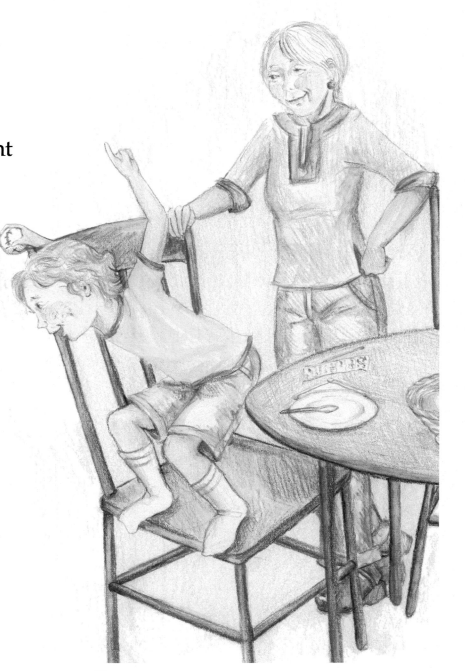

Grandma followed Teddy into the living room and sat down on the sofa. Elaine was sitting next to her Grandfather. "I wanted Grandpa to know he was not alone, so I've been holding his hand." "This is a nice little girl, Mary." Grandpa Jack was clearly enjoying Elaine's company.

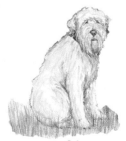

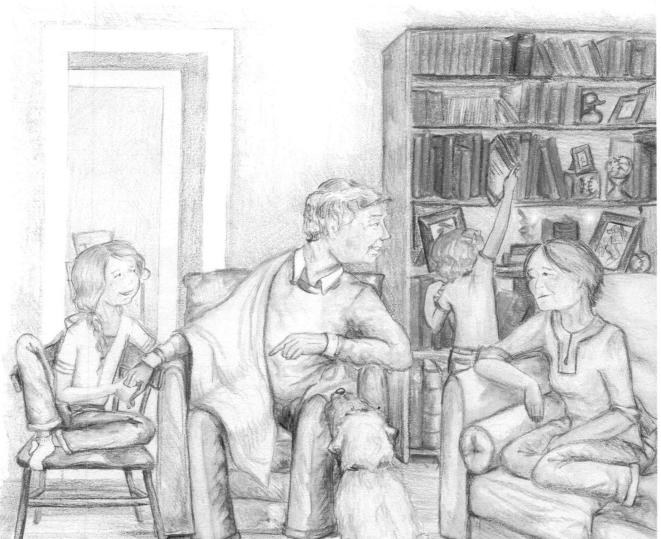

"We've been playing a game—I squeeze Grandpa's hand and he squeezes mine right back. And, I promised Grandpa that next week I'll bring my seashell collection so we can pretend we're at the beach!" "You've really got the idea now," Grandma said with amusement.

Teddy found the book he wanted and settled at Grandpa's feet. "I'm going to read you a story Grandpa—it's about Willie Mays, a great baseball player."

1954 The Catch

It was the top of the eighth inning in the first game of the series—Mays took off, as did the base runners, thinking it couldn't be caught. He did catch it, over his shoulder. Immediately, he whipped around and sent the ball off to the infield, kept the runners from scoring and one runner off the diamond…it's entirely possible that the Indians would have won the World Series if Mays hadn't made the catch.

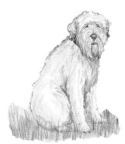

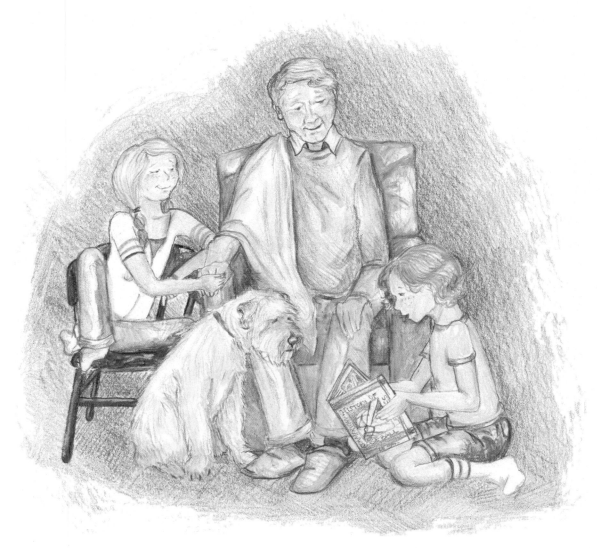

Teddy looked up at Grandpa Jack, who was listening intently.
"Good story," Grandpa said in a quiet voice. "I thought you'd like
it." Teddy said. "Next week we can play a little catch together if
you want to. Don't worry though, Grandpa—I'll be your coach."
Grandpa Jack nodded his head and smiled.

When it was time to go home, the children climbed into Grandpa's chair to say goodbye. "Group Hug!" Elaine and Teddy exclaimed.

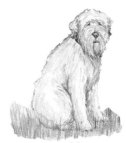

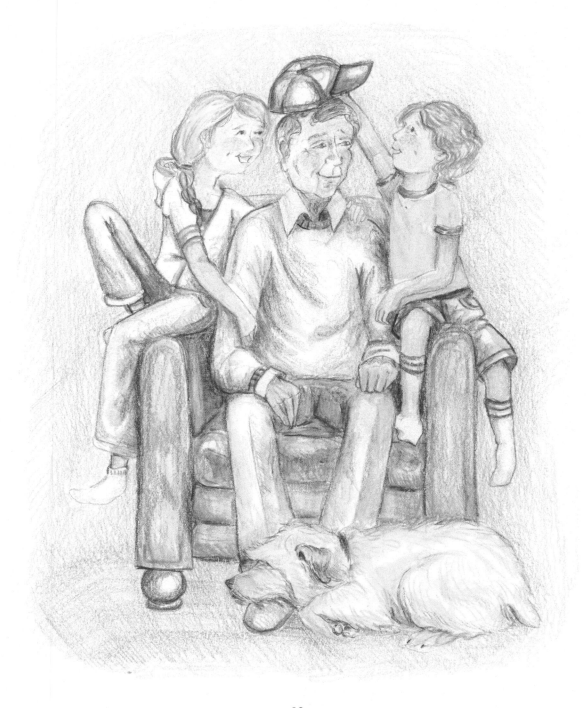

As the children cozied up to Grandpa Jack, loud snoring sounds erupted from the sofa. "I guess Grandma Mary's pretty good at sawing wood too!" Elaine grinned. And with that, they all snuggled together with a little chuckle.

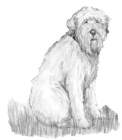

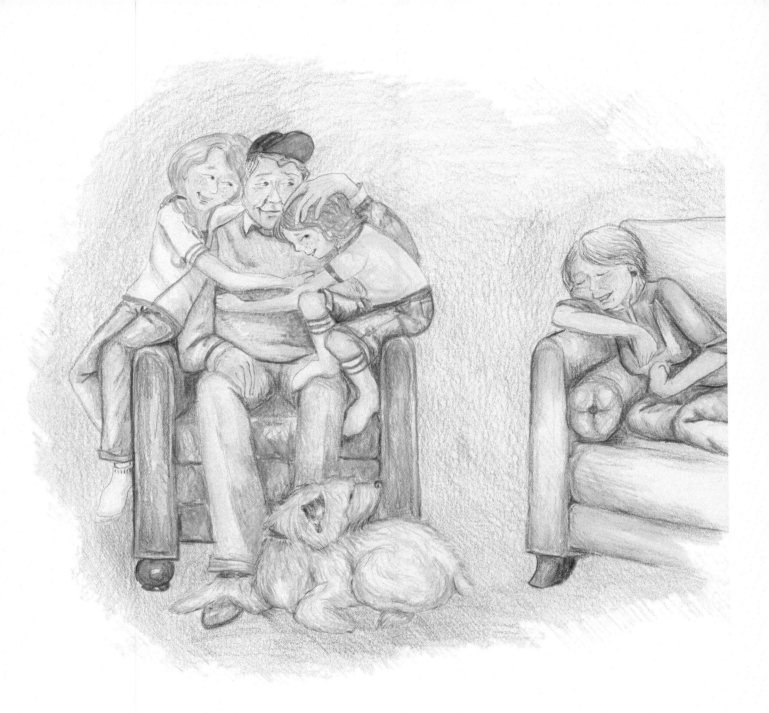

Your List:
What Makes You Feel Loved?

A Note to Children:

If you've read this story, chances are you may already know how hard it is to watch a grandparent or parent become confused and forgetful. What a person can do and enjoy depends on the memory disease they have and how long they've had it. A person's memory can change quickly or slowly. It's important to know that one thing never changes for your loved one with memory loss: your ability to brighten their day by spending time with them!

Think about the abilities your grandparent or parent still has. Think about which senses, (hearing, taste, touch, sight and smell) are in good shape. Focusing on what a person CAN do helps create small, important moments of happiness in their day. Learning about your loved one's hobbies and jobs, and the time in history when they were growing up will help you figure out meaningful things you can do together. Sometimes people mostly enjoy quiet activities or just having you nearby to keep them company. Also, it can be helpful to wear a nametag when you're with them.

Here's a special tip: Animals, music and nature are like magic for most people living with memory loss. Your loved one may need help to make these special things a part of their day. For example, if there is a new kitten or puppy in the neighborhood, share it with your grandparent or parent. If your family member can't go outside, bring the outdoors to them. People love seeing and touching colorful fall leaves, spring flowers and fresh vegetables. They love the smell of freshly cut grass and soft, cold snow. You can even make an indoor snowman in the winter!

If you try to do something with your grandparent or parent and it doesn't go well, don't worry; he or she is probably just having a hard day. You can't force an activity, but you can always try again when they are feeling better.

The following pages have communication tips, book and website suggestions, and activity ideas to help you stay connected with your loved one. Many activities can be adapted for someone in a bed or wheelchair. Be creative and keep it REAL! You will find the heart has a memory of its own. TM ☺

Resources for Children and Families

Tips for Talking to Someone Who has Memory Loss

*Eye contact shows you're Listening

*Gentle touch can be Calming

*Waiting for answers brings Surprises

*Repeating their words makes Sense

*Kind words are Comforting

*a Calm voice works Wonders

*a Calm body will be Copied

*Seeing you talk is Helpful

*Listening is Appreciated

*a Smile will touch the Heart

*Feelings need to be Noticed!

Memory/Activity Scale For Children ©2010 Theresa Matocha
(Use the 3 Categories Below to Understand Your Loved One's Abilities)

Activity Ideas	A Little Forgetful Knows your face Knows your name Can do daily tasks (eats/dresses w/o help)	Mostly Forgetful Sometimes knows face Sometimes knows name Does some task w/o help (can eat/dress w/help)	Very Forgetful Rarely knows your face Rarely knows your name Needs help w/all tasks
Nature/ Outdoors	*Rake Leaves *Weed Garden *Visit aquarium/zoo	*Brush Dog *Pick Berries *Moon/Star Gaze	*Watch Birds *Touch Fruit/Leaves *Sit Under a Tree
Cozy Time	*Make a Memory Box *Read a Story Together *Look at Family Photos	*Trade Hand Massages *Read a Story Out Loud *Snuggle with Music	*Snuggle in a Blanket *Gently Brush Hair *Share a Cup of Tea
Games	*Scrabble/Pictionary *Checkers/Chess/Cards *Catch/Ping Pong	*Name that Tune/Bird *Ring Toss/Checkers *Finish the Rhyme e.g. a stitch in time.......	If able: Recite Proverbs e.g. a rolling stone........ *If able: Clap to Music
Just For Fun	*Visit an Art Museum *Dance to Music *Paint a Canvas	*Sort Old Jewelry/Ties *Paint a Canvas *Make Theme Books (cats/trees/birds)	*Share a 'Touch Box' (soft fabrics/tree bark) *Listen to Music *Hold a Gentle Animal

Activity Books:

Bell, Virginia et al. <u>Best Friends Book of Alzheimer's Activities</u>. Maryland: Health Professions Press, 2002.

Burdick, Lydia. <u>Wishing on a Star: A read Aloud Book for Memory Challenged Adults</u>. Maryland: Health Professions Press, 2009.

Camp, Cameron J. ed. <u>Montessori-Based Activities for Persons with Dementia</u>.Vol. I. Maryland: Health Professions Press, 2001.

<u>Montessori-Based Activities for Persons with Dementia.</u> Vol.II. Maryland: Health Professions Press, 2006.

Lebul Ziegler, Rae Lynn. <u>Let's Look Together, An Interactive Picture Book for People with Alzheimer's Dementia and Other Types of Dementia.</u> Maryland: Health Professions Press, 2009.

Bruce, Hank and Jill Folk-Tomi. <u>Alzheimer's with a Green Thumb; Gardening as Therapy for People with Dementia and Their Families.</u> New Mexico: Petals and Pages Press, 2015.

Story Books:

Bahr, M. The Memory Box. Illinois: L.A. Whitman & Company, 1992.

[for 7-11 year olds; in the early stages of memory loss, grandpa helps the family create a special memory box as a way to cope with coming changes]

Gardner, Linda and Sarah Langford, Emily Jiang, ed. Grandfather's Story Cloth. California: Shen's Books, 2008.

[for 4-8 year olds; a revered family elder and his young grandson share memories using a beautiful woven story cloth]

Kukugawa, Frances. Wordsworth Dances theWaltz. Haiwaii: Watermark Publishing, 2007.

[for 7-10 year olds; Wordsworth the poet mouse helps his family understand that Grandma still loves laughing, dancing and family time despite her memory loss]

McIntyre, Connie and Louise McIntyre. Flowers for Grandpa Dan: A Gentle Story To Help Children Understand Alzheimer's Disease. Missouri: Thumbprint Press, 2005.

[for 7-11 year olds; a little boy learns to cope with his Grandfather's memory loss]

Simard, Joyce. The Magic Tape Recorder. Prague: Joyce Simard Publishing and Czech Republic Publishing, 2007.

[for children of all ages to help them understand memory loss and their role as helpers]

Websites for Children and Families:

https://abesgarden.org

[resources related to memory/senior life communities that focus on brain health, wellness and purposeful living.]

http://www.alz.org/help-support/resources/kids-teens

[sponsored by the Alzheimer's Association-comprehensive resources for young children, teens, parents and teachers]

www.angelfire.com/ma/alrac/kidsad.html

[link to dementia info page for younger kids—explains dementia and offers ideas for interacting with a loved one]

http://faculty.washington.edu/chudler/neurok.html

[website for kids about neuroscience—good section on memory and related issues]

http://kidshealth.org/kid/health_problems/brain/memory.html

[section for older kids and teens—good straight forward info about how memories are formed and the various causes of dementia]

www.nccdp.org

[website for The National Council of Certified Dementia Practitioners.
Excellent source of information for every aspect of dementia care; from activities to educational tools as well as links to other important sites for caregivers]

https://www.thehearthstoneinstitute.org

[pioneers of a hopeful and positive approach to memory care; information re: caregiver training, research and other resources.]

About the Author

Theresa Matocha holds a Master's degree in social work and completed a gerontology internship at Baylor College of Medicine's Geriatric Clinic and Diagnostic Center. She is a licensed clinical social worker, certified dementia practitioner and former instructor with the National Council of Certified Dementia Practitioners, a certified clinical trauma professional and psychotherapist. As a former program director of a fifty-resident special care unit -she was inspired by the positive impact authentic sensory experiences, dignified activities and emotional validation had on people with varied forms of memory-loss. With this book, she hopes to spread awareness of the person-centered, strengths-based model of dementia care and its ability to enhance life quality within every stage of memory loss. Theresa's professional profile can be viewed via **psychologytoday.com**

About the Illustrator

Lilli Stein studied theatre and Russian language at Middlebury College in Middlebury, Vermont. She is an actress and artist living in Brooklyn, New York. To view more of her work you can visit her profile in IMDb or at **lillistein.com**

Printed in the United States
by Baker & Taylor Publisher Services